THE MEDITERRANEAN DASH DIET COOKBOOK FOR BEGINNERS

The Best Tasty Recipes To Change your Lifestyle and Improve your Health.

Table of Contents

Introduction 6

Chapter 1.   What is the DASH Diet? 7

What Does DASH Mean? 7

Electrolytes 7

What about Weight Loss and Diabetes? 9

What Is a Good Blood Pressure Reading? 9

Dietary Approaches to Stop Hypertension 12

Causes of High Blood Pressure 12

Chapter 2.   The DASH Diet Food List 15

Fruits 16

Meat 20

Beans, Nuts, and Seeds 23

Salad Dressing, Oils, and Mayo 24

Sweets 24

Alcohol 25

Foods to Avoid on the DASH Diet 27

Chapter 3.   Breakfast and Smoothies Recipes 29

Orange-Blueberry Muffin 29

Baked Ginger Oatmeal with Pear Topping 30

Greek-Style Veggie Omelet 32

Sweet Potatoes with Coconut Flakes 33

Flaxseed & Banana Smoothie 35

Fruity Tofu Smoothie..36

French Toast with Applesauce 37

Banana-Peanut Butter 'n Greens Smoothie.............................38

Baking Powder Biscuits 39

Oatmeal Banana Pancakes with Walnuts................................41

Creamy Oats, Greens & Blueberry Smoothie 42

Banana & Cinnamon Oatmeal...43

Bagels Made Healthy..44

Chapter 4.   Lunch Recipes..46

Kushari 46

Bulgur with Tomatoes and Chickpeas.....................................48

Mackerel Maccheroni 50

Maccheroni with Cherry Tomatoes and Anchovies.................52

Lemon and Shrimp Risotto..54

Spaghetti with Clams..56

Greek Fish Soup 58

Venere Rice with Shrimp..60

Pennette with Salmon and Vodka..62

Seafood Carbonara 64

Garganelli with Zucchini Pesto and Shrimp...........................67

Salmon Risotto...69

Chapter 5.   Dinner Recipes 72

Stuffed Bell Peppers 72

Stuffed Eggplants with Goat Cheese... 74

Korma Curry 76

Zucchini Bars 78

Mushroom Soup 80

Stuffed Portobello Mushrooms.. 81

Lettuce Salad 83

Lemon Garlic Salmon.. 85

Chickpea Curry 86

Instant Pot Chicken Thighs with Olives and Capers................... 89

Instant Pot salmon 91

Instant Pot Mac N' Cheese.. 92

Chapter 6.   Dessert Recipes 94

The Most Elegant Parsley Soufflé Ever....................................... 94

Fennel and Almond Bites... 95

Feisty Coconut Fudge.. 96

No Bake Cheesecake.. 98

Easy Chia Seed Pumpkin Pudding... 99

Lovely Blueberry Pudding.. 101

Decisive Lime and Strawberry Popsicle.................................... 102

Ravaging Blueberry Muffin 103

The Coconut Loaf.. 105

Fresh Figs with Walnuts and Ricotta.. 106

Authentic Medjool Date Truffles.. 107

Tasty Mediterranean Peanut Almond Butter Popcorns 109

Just A Minute Worth Muffin 110

Hearty Almond Bread 111

Introduction

The Mediterranean DASH diet is designed to help you lower your blood pressure, improve cardiac health, reduce the risk of cancer and type 2 diabetes, and, in some cases, lose weight. The Mediterranean diet is based on eating, cooking, and other lifestyle factors that focus on an abundance of whole foods. The DASH diet was created to avoid hypertension through the intake of some nutrients and others' elimination. These two diets overlap in many areas, but merging them fully creates a powerful duo that is sustainable—and delicious—for the long term. It's no wonder they've been the top two diets, as ranked by U.S. News & World Report, for many years running.

The combination of the two diets creates an exclusive method to the DASH diet that is extremely flexible, packed with vegetarian and pastry options, and it makes cooking at home or eating out easy and doable. Once you understand the basics and start building your recipe arsenal, customizing your favorite dishes will become second nature. You never have to be afraid of running out of recipe ideas!

As someone who has a deep love for both food and health, I've filled this book with satisfying dishes rooted in the flavorful culinary traditions of Greece, Italy, and Spain, among others, and included tips to make committing to this nutritionally balanced way of eating as easy as possible. I hope you'll find the information in this book and the recipes as useful and tasty as I do. Enough of the pep talk. It's time to get started. Let's find out what the Mediterranean DASH diet is all about, how and why it was developed, and how you can use it to improve your health!

Chapter 1.   What is the DASH Diet?

We will explore the history of the DASH diet. First, we'll learn why the DASH diet was developed and the theory behind it. Then we'll look at how early trials of the DASH diet developed and the results. We'll talk about the general benefits of the DASH diet, which we will explore in more detail in later chapters.

What Does DASH Mean?

DASH simply means Dietary Approaches to Stop Hypertension. Hypertension or having a high BP is a common but very serious health problem that was once called the "silent killer." Doing damage to blood vessels and key body organs can lead to ill health and even death. Some of the high blood pressure victims have been world-famous—U.S. President Franklin Delano Roosevelt was among them, sadly living in a time just before the first pharmaceutical treatments for and understanding of hypertension came about. He died in 1945 near the end of the Second World War, and some of the first effective treatments for high blood pressure were developed just a few years later, in the 1950s.

Electrolytes

We don't want to make your eyes glaze over by going too deeply into the science, but a few basic facts will help you understand high BP and the DASH diet. First, we need to know what an electrolyte is; simply put, it's a substance in your body that is "ionized." In other words, it carries an electrical charge. Electrolytes are very important when it comes to the basic functionality of the body's systems. In particular, they are involved in nerve function or neurotransmission, and they help regulate how the blood vessels behave.

The main electrolytes related to nerve function and the function of your blood vessels are:

- Sodium

- Potassium

- Calcium

- Magnesium

We don't need to know the details, but we can understand how these work in the body in the following way:

- Sodium tightens your blood vessels, or in another way, tends to increase blood pressure. Sodium is also closely associated with fluid retention.

- Potassium, calcium, and magnesium are associated with relaxing the blood vessels or putting another way to lower blood pressure.

- Calcium also contributes to lowering blood pressure.

Sodium, potassium, magnesium, and calcium are all important for the heart muscle's proper function. For example, a magnesium or potassium deficiency can lead to palpitations or problems with heart rhythms. Severe deficiencies of any of these minerals can even lead to heart arrhythmias that are so drastic they can be fatal.

It's important to understand that sodium (or salt, which is how we get sodium through our diets) is not an evil or bad thing. You must have salt in your diet—without sodium, your body would not function properly. In fact, recently, a woman in Israel suffered major brain damage following a fruit juice only diet. Doctors explained that it was the lack of salt, which caused her health crisis. Fruit has lots of potassium and magnesium but very little sodium. For more info on the story, see "Fruit juice diet sends a woman to the hospital with brain damage."

The article about the fruit juice diet makes something clear—the balance between sodium, potassium, calcium, and magnesium is what's important.

What about Weight Loss and Diabetes?

As we'll see, the DASH diet strictly limits servings and portions but does it in a very easy-to-follow way. By regulating overall food intake and specific numbers of servings for each food group, the diet naturally leads to weight loss for those who need it. As a side benefit, the focus on whole grains and lean proteins helps those who are pre-diabetic or even those who have full-blown diabetes. These issues will be explored in more detail in later chapters.

What Is a Good Blood Pressure Reading?

Many folks know that having high blood pressure is bad for their health, but they aren't clear on the details. So let's lay them out here.

For the most part, doctors consider healthy blood pressure to be around 120/80 or lower. Obviously, it can't be drastically lower than this; very low blood pressure can cause lots of problems on its own such as making you pass out. However, some doctors are taking a harder line, suggesting that your blood pressure should be 115/75 to be considered "normal." However, it's not entirely clear that having it that low is consequential for health.

When your blood pressure inches upward into higher ranges, you're considered to have so-called "pre-hypertension." This is a range at which there aren't going to be any short-term health consequences (and maybe none ever) but that you're in danger of running into future trouble. It's also considered a range where you're more likely to get things under control by making lifestyle changes rather than having to go on medication. For systolic blood pressure, the pre-hypertension range is generally considered to be 120-129 mm Hg. For diastolic blood pressure, the range is 80-89 mm Hg.

For all blood pressures higher than these values, medical professionals divide them into three ranges. These are:

- Stage 1: this is between 140/90 and 150/99. Whether or not you will be placed on medication or not may vary by the doctor, but most will probably put you on a mild or low-dose blood pressure medication.

- Stage 2: this is considered far more serious with implications for overall health. The range here is 160/100 and higher.

- Emergency: if your blood pressure tops 180/110, then this is considered a medical emergency, and a trip to a hospital is warranted.

Doctors may also consider the range between diastolic and systolic blood pressure. The difference between the two is called pulse pressure. So if you have a blood pressure of 135/90, your pulse pressure is 135 mm Hg

– 90 mm Hg = 45 mm Hg. Since 120/80 is still considered the ideal blood pressure, you can see that a pulse pressure of about 40 mm Hg is what would be considered healthy.

A high or low pulse pressure can indicate problems, especially for patients over the age of 60. If the pulse pressure is high, this indicates a high risk of future heart attack or stroke. This holds more strongly for men but is true generally. If pulse pressure is greater than 60 mm Hg, the patient is considered to be at higher risk of a future heart attack. However, a high pulse pressure may also indicate other health problems related to the cardiovascular system, like leaky heart valves.

Low pulse pressure can indicate health problems as well. That can indicate that the heart is not working properly, has become weakened.

While a pulse pressure of 40 mm Hg is a good value when we are talking about blood pressures in the normal range, it can't be taken in isolation. If you had a blood pressure of 170/130, your pulse pressure would also be 40 mm Hg, but a patient with a blood pressure of 170/130 is at a lot higher risk than one with a blood pressure of 130/90 or even someone with larger pulse pressure but lower overall values, like 140/90 which would be a pulse pressure of 50 mm Hg.

High pulse pressure can be caused by damage to the aorta, which is the main artery supplying the heart. If you have heart disease, which means plaque buildup from fatty calcium deposits in your arteries, they stiffen. Stiffened arteries don't respond to changes in the force of pumping blood as well as normal arteries, leading to higher pulse pressure.

Blood pressure medications not only reduce overall blood pressure but may also help lower pulse pressure.

Dietary Approaches to Stop Hypertension

Causes of High Blood Pressure

High blood pressure is one of the most serious health problems worldwide, with up to a billion people estimated to have high blood pressure. It's more acute in developed countries, and when we examine possible causes of high blood pressure, the reasons why become clear. In the United States, it's estimated that about 50 million people are suffering from high blood pressure. The actual number is unknown, and it's often called "the silent killer". The reason is that someone can appear to be completely healthy and yet have high blood pressure. Their body may look fine from the outside, but internally it's being destroyed minute by minute.

Some of the most common causes that have been identified include:

- Smoking: cigarette smoking, in particular, due to the fact people get more nicotine in their system, has been strongly identified as an environmental risk factor for developing high blood pressure.

- Weight gain/obesity: not all overweight people have high blood pressure, but it's clear that being overweight significantly increases your risk of developing it. The heavier you get, the higher the risk.

- Sedentary lifestyle: exercise definitely counteracts hypertension. It helps keep the blood vessels flexible and responsive and helps keep the heart in shape. Someone who has cardiovascular fitness has a lower resting heart rate, and their heart pumps with a healthier level of force, so the blood pressure is reduced compared to what it would be otherwise. In contrast, people who don't exercise raise their risk of developing high blood pressure, especially if they have a family history.

- Race: African Americans are more prone to high blood pressure than other groups. However, bear in mind that all racial and ethnic groups have plenty of risk of high blood pressure and its victims include people of all races and from every country across the globe.

- Kidney disease: the kidneys are closely tied to the healthy maintenance of blood sugar. They help regulate the amount of fluid and salt in the body. When you are suffering from kidney disease, they may not function as well, and this may lead to fluid and sodium retention, which can cause high blood pressure.

- Age: simply getting older raises risk, although we would never call high blood pressure "normal." However, as you get older, things don't work as well (you knew that, right?). If your joints are stiffening, you can bet your arteries are as well. So even though you may be reasonably healthy overall, simply getting older raises your risk of developing some level of high blood pressure. There is some debate about whether older people need to be put under the same standards as to what constitutes a hypertension diagnosis or not, but a general rule applies. You're better off if your blood pressure is below 140/100.

- Nutritional deficiencies: by now, you're an expert—nutritional deficiencies of potassium and magnesium can lead to high blood pressure and other health problems like heart palpitations and muscle cramps.

- Excessive salt in the diet: we've reviewed this one already— salt causes your body to retain fluid, and it promotes contraction of blood vessels, among other things.

The DASH diet provides an opportunity to address several items on this list. It reduces salt in the diet and addresses the nutritional deficiencies in potassium and magnesium. By consuming large amounts of fruits and vegetables along with a low-fat diet, you'll find that your risk of kidney disease drops as well. Controlling weight can also reduce the risks of developing high blood pressure.

Chapter 2. The DASH Diet Food List

Now let's take a deep dive into foods you can eat and foods you should either consume in moderation or avoid completely while following the DASH diet. Remember, the starting point of the DASH diet is to limit sodium consumption. If this is your first time on the DASH diet, it's advised that you follow the standard DASH diet, which limits sodium consumption to 2,300 mg per day. To be honest, you don't need to be completely religious about it. If you end up eating 2,500 mg of sodium per day, you're still OK, and if you eat 2,200 one day and 2,800 the next, you're fine too, if your average for the entire week comes in around 2,300-2,500 mg per day. As long as you're staying well below the average American who is consuming 3,400 mg per day of sodium, you're probably doing well at meeting your overall goals.

If you are going on this diet because of high blood pressure, and you find that hitting close to the 2,300 mg average but not seeing any results, then you can try the low sodium version of the diet. This limits sodium intake to 1,500 mg per day. Be sure to discuss these issues with your doctor before doing so.

Remember that the DASH diet's main components are fruits and vegetables, whole grains, lean meats, and low-fat dairy. The DASH diet doesn't worry about calorie counting or weighing food; just refer back to the DASH diet food pyramid to get portion counts and sizes. We're going to look at a few items in detail; since the DASH diet is so focused on getting the right amounts of potassium, sodium, magnesium, and calcium, it helps to have some awareness of what some foods actually contain.

Fruits

Fruits tend to contain large amounts of potassium and magnesium and very low sodium. As a result, they play a central role in the DASH diet. For example, let's look at the nutrition content of a medium-sized apple:

- Calories: 95

- Sodium: 2 mg

- Potassium: 195 mg

- Magnesium: 2% of the daily value

- Calcium: 1% of the daily value

We picked an apple as our first example on purpose. You remember that in Japan, it was noticed that people in regions where large amounts of apples were consumed had much lower rates of stroke. By looking at an apple's nutrition facts, we see virtually no sodium in an apple at all but a fair amount of potassium. So eating an apple a day really does keep the doctor away, in the sense that it's going to help rebalance your electrolytes by adding potassium practically all by itself. Let's check the nutrition facts for a large orange:

- Calories: 87

- Sodium: 0 mg

- Potassium: 333 mg

- Magnesium: 4% of the daily value

- Calcium: 7% of the daily value

Orange is even better for the DASH diet than an apple—it's got a lot more potassium and no sodium at all while giving us slightly higher amounts of calcium and magnesium.

The DASH diet was developed way back in 1992, during a time when fat was the enemy. If you've been paying attention, you've probably noticed that the attitude about fat is shifting. When it comes to certain fat types, like the omega-3 oils in fish and the monounsaturated fat in olive oil, the attitude has completely transformed. Now, these types of fats are viewed as healthy and as healthy, perhaps as vital to good health, particularly for the cardiovascular system.

With that in mind, although it's not generally discussed within the context of the DASH diet – I would like to introduce you to the avocado. Those who are interested in following the "Mediterranean" version of the DASH diet will certainly be interested in avocados. Like olive oil, avocado oil is primarily monounsaturated fat, which is believed to reduce inflammation. The only issue with avocados is being aware of the calorie content—since they are a fat-based fruit, they pack more calories than most fruits. A suggestion is to eat a ½ of an avocado instead of a whole one, and of course, there is wide variation in size, so you can reap the benefits while opting for smaller avocados with fewer calories. Let's look at the nutritional content of a medium-sized avocado:

- Calories: 332

- Fat: 29 grams (20 g is monounsaturated fat)

- Sodium: 14 mg

- Potassium: 975 mg

- Magnesium: 14% of the daily value

- Calcium: 2% of the daily value

If you take a close look, you'll notice that avocados are PACKING in potassium. If you're shooting for 4,700 mg of potassium per day, then avocado is a good start, as recommended by the DASH diet. Moreover, avocados also contain 14% of daily-recommended magnesium. Avocados are also loaded with dietary fiber. One avocado provides 40% of the fiber you need each day.

While the DASH diet allows the consumption of frozen and dried fruits, you may think carefully about consuming these foods. This issue comes up because, once again, the DASH diet was originally developed in 1992. In a nutritional sense, it almost seems like the dark ages. At that time, there wasn't the awareness of the problems with sugar consumption that there is now. The problem with frozen and dried fruit is that they contain concentrated sugar. You will want to avoid sugar and make sure you consume the whole fruit with all the fiber. The fiber helps slow digestion and reduces blood sugar spikes, along with all the harm that comes with them. For that reason, although fruit juice is permitted daily on the DASH diet, we recommend only consuming it in moderation, if at all. This advice is especially important for people who have pre-diabetes or who have diabetes. In that case, you're far better off eating an avocado than you are drinking orange juice or indulging in dried fruit snacks.

Peach is also an excellent choice for fruit. It's low calorie and high potassium.

- Calories: 59

- Sodium: 0 mg

- Potassium: 285 mg

- Magnesium: 3% of the daily value

- Calcium: 0% of daily value

Here is a complete list of fruits you can choose from to round out your first month on the DASH diet:

- Apple

- Avocado

- Banana

- Blackberries

- Blueberries

- Cantaloupe

- Cherries

- Dates

- Grapes

- Kiwi

- Mango

- Nectarines

- Oranges

- Peach

- Raspberries

- Strawberries

- Tomatoes

Yes, don't forget that tomatoes are fruits even though they kind of seem like vegetables. Berries are an excellent choice because they are packed with nutrients but have a low sugar content and glycemic index when compared to most fruits. We could list far more fruits than we have here, but we're going to limit our food lists because we want to keep things as simple as possible for people starting with the DASH diet.

While dairy products do contain significant amounts of sodium, they are perfectly healthy since they contain more potassium. They also provide important calcium and some magnesium as well. If osteoporosis is an issue that you're worried about, having a cup of milk and a serving of yogurt each day should be an important part of your diet. In fact, you should probably consume the fully allowed 3 portions, either by adding some cheese or a second serving of milk or yogurt if that describes your situation.

Meat

When it comes to meat, the DASH diet is fairly flexible, but it does take the perspective of a low-fat diet. As a result, low-fat cuts of meat and poultry without skin are the order of the day. Since fish fat is deemed healthy, you can eat fatty fish serving without worrying about it.

A serving size of meat is 3 oz.., but to be that strict all the time is probably beyond most people. So you might aim for between 3-5 oz.. per servings. When craving foods like hamburgers or sausage, you can still enjoy them if you look for low-fat alternatives made out of meats like turkey and chicken.

Poultry should be consumed without the skin. That means chicken wings are out, but skinless chicken breast and skinless chicken thighs are in. Turkey's legs and thighs have too much fat; you should stick to the skinless breast when it comes to turkey. Duck is a popular poultry item, but it's best avoided on the DASH diet because duck has a high-fat content relative to chicken and turkey.

Lean cuts of beef can be enjoyed on a moderate basis. That doesn't mean that you have to eat beef every day. There is no specific recommendation, but you should probably aim for once a week or less. When selecting beef, aim for lean cuts like sirloin. Ground beef can be eaten from time to time as long as you get the lowest fat variety available (look for 96%). Pork sausage should be avoided. When consuming other pork products, avoid ribs and aim for lean pork loins or pork chops trimmed with fat. Many experts consider pork a "red meat," even though the pork industry used to try selling itself as the "other white meat."

You should select sirloin, chuck shoulder, top loin, round steaks, and roasts for beef. Fatty cuts like prime rib, rib eye, porterhouse, T-bone, and New York strip should be avoided.

Exotic meats can find their way on the DASH diet menu to make your meals more interesting and varied. For example, consider elk, which is available in stores like Whole Foods and Sprouts. Elk is similar to beef in taste and texture (we are talking farm-raised elk here), but it's extremely lean. Many cuts of elk steak are only 3% fat.

Other exotic meats—of the farm-raised variety—you can consider to include kangaroo and ostrich. These are also both red meat and extremely lean.

Processed meats should be avoided at all costs. So you should not be consuming salami, pepperoni, hot dogs, or even bacon, even if they are low-fat varieties. The main reason is that you must avoid the high sodium content of these meats.

When it comes to fish, you can consume virtually everything as long as you don't overdo the portions. Feel free to eat salmon, tuna, sardines, mackerel, swordfish, and trout to your desired level, up to 2 servings per day. You can also consume lean fish like cod and sole provided that it's not breaded unless the coating is made from whole grain flour. The health benefits of fish oil, when consumed in whole fish, are indisputable. The only fish that is really prohibited are canned anchovies and salted cod. As you probably know, anchovies are packed in salt and on a diet that is based on low sodium intake, anchovies don't make the cut.

Being the leanest proteins on the planet, other types of seafood are definitely acceptable on the DASH diet. This includes shrimp, scallops, oysters, crab, and lobster. However, remember that your consumption of "butter" is limited to margarine and in small amounts. If you do eat lobster with butter (use a substitute like margarine, we are speaking colloquially here), make sure you know how much you're using. No doubt it's going to exceed the specified amounts allowed by the DASH diet per day—but you could make up for it the following day by consuming reduced servings from the oil, salad dressing, and mayo category.

Beans, Nuts, and Seeds

Next up, we have the beans, nuts, and seeds category. If you're seeking out a low-fat diet, beans are often highly recommended because they have low fat, they are high-quality protein, and they have lots of fiber. If you're a vegan or vegetarian, you can substitute them for the 0-2 servings of meat per day. However, if you're a meat-eater, you'll be limiting your servings of beans, nuts, and seeds, to one serving per day. This category also includes so-called "legumes" such as lentils, peas, and soybeans. Peanuts are also technically a legume, although most of us think of them as nuts.

You have the option of selecting nuts or seeds for your daily serving. Nuts and seeds have high-fat content, which is why they aren't recommended in large amounts. However, note that nuts have lots of healthy monounsaturated fat and also contain large amounts of potassium and magnesium.

It's understandable why nuts and seeds are limited to one serving daily since they contain a lot of fat and, therefore, they're calorie-dense. However, it's not really clear why the DASH diet designers would limit the consumption of beans. Beans are rich in certain vitamins, provide a practically zero fat source of protein, and also contain large amounts of needed dietary fiber. What's not to love about beans in the context of a healthy diet? In our view, you can increase bean consumption if you substitute it for meat. Studies show that people who eat nuts on a daily basis have a significantly reduced risk of heart disease. So it makes more sense to eat a serving of nuts once per day, and then when you want to eat beans, substitute them for a serving of meat.

Salad Dressing, Oils, and Mayo

The DASH diet is very restrictive when it comes to these items. You're only allowed 2-3 servings per day. Examples include:

- Canola oil

- Olive oil

- Mayo

- Low-fat or fat-free salad dressings

Soft margarine, but consider smart balance, which is hard but a very healthy alternative.

Sweets

Finally, we come to the topic of sweets. As we discussed earlier, "sweets" in the DASH diet might not meet your sweets concept. They aren't talking about cake, pie, and ice cream, although they allow small amounts of sugar, honey, and syrup. For the DASH dieter, a sweet consists of frozen yogurt or a serving of yogurt with fruit. It's not entirely clear why frozen yogurt is permitted while ice cream is not. Our take is you can eat certain ice cream varieties—using the limited five serving per week guide. But be careful and read labels. Let's compare the nutrition for a ½ cup serving of frozen yogurt to a ½ cup serving of vanilla ice cream. According to a search on nutrition facts on Google, for the yogurt we have:

- Calories: 114

- Fat grams: 4

- Sugar: 17

For vanilla ice cream, we find:

- Calories: 137

- Fat grams: 7

- Sugar: 14

Since we're only having at most five servings per week, that extra 23 calories and 3 grams of fat from vanilla ice cream are not going to matter at all. The increased fat in the vanilla ice cream is matched by more sugar in the yogurt. You could argue that you should have low-fat yogurt, but you can get low-fat vanilla ice cream as well. So in our view, as long as you carefully measure your servings and only consume up to five servings per week, some real ice cream isn't going to throw off your diet.

And if you think it is, then buy the ice cream for a time and see if things improve.

Alcohol

Alcohol is not explicitly discussed on the DASH diet, but it's so important we better mention it for those readers who are adults and like to drink. The general thought is that alcohol can be consumed in moderation while following the DASH diet. That means for men, 2-3 drinks per day and for women 1-2 drinks per day. You need to be aware that alcohol does add extra calories, especially if you're imbibing mixed drinks that can be loaded up with sugar, syrups, and cream. It's best to stick to straight liquor or, even better, beer and wine. While the DASH diet is not a calorie-counting diet, you need to have some awareness if you drink alcohol. That means cutting some calories somewhere else. For example, you might consider wine as a serving of fruit, and quite frankly, it is. Let's look at the nutrition of red wine:

- Calories: 125

- Sodium: 6 mg

- Potassium: 187 mg

- Magnesium: 4% of the daily value

- Calcium: 1% of the daily value

That nutrition profile isn't much different from that seen for many fruits, and that really isn't surprising since wine is made out of grapes, but I doubt that many readers have thought of drinking wine to get some extra potassium.

Beer also provides some potassium, but it also contains more sodium. It also provides a small amount of magnesium. Beer is starchier, so if you are going to drink beer, you might consider substituting it for one serving of grains. Calling beer a vegetable might be too much of a stretch.

One concern regarding alcohol is that consuming alcohol can increase blood pressure in some people. You'll need to check this out for yourself and see if you're sensitive to that.

Foods to Avoid on the DASH Diet

Although we have talked about many foods to avoid, we thought we should gather them here for the sake of reference. When it comes to fruits and vegetables, there are no foods that are prohibited. So we'll start with grains.

Prohibited grains:

- White bread.

- White rice.

- White pasta.

- White flour, refined.

- White hamburger buns and hot dog rolls.

- Sourdough bread.

- French bread.

- Any cereal with added sugar.

- Breakfast "cereals" made from refined grains and flour.

- Any snacks containing sugar.

- Any snack that is high in sodium (for example, Triscuits may be whole grain, but they are high in salt). Get a low-sodium variety).

- Any snacks that contain Trans fats.

However, there are some dairy products to avoid:

- Butter and ghee

- Heavy cream

- Whipped cream

- Half-and-Half

- Buttermilk

- Egg nog

Chapter 3.   Breakfast and Smoothies Recipes

Orange-Blueberry Muffin

Preparation Time: 10 minutes

Cooking Time: 10-25 minutes

Servings: 12

Difficulty Level: Average

Ingredients:

- 1 3/4 cups of all-purpose flour

- 1/3 cup of sugar

- 2 1/2 teaspoons of baking powder

- 1/2 teaspoon of baking soda

- 1/2 teaspoon of salt

- 1/2 teaspoon of ground cinnamon

- 3/4 cup of milk, fat-free (skim)

- 1/4 cup of butter

- 1 egg, large, lightly beaten

- 3 tablespoons of thawed orange juice concentrate

- 1 teaspoon of vanilla

- 3/4 cup of fresh blueberries

Directions:

1. Ready your oven to 400 ° F. Follow steps 2 to 5 of the Buckwheat Apple-Raisin Muffin recipe. Fill up the muffin cups ¾-full of the mixture and bake for 20 to 25 minutes. Let it cool for 5 minutes and serve warm.

Nutrition (for 100g):

- Calories 149

- Fat 5g

- Carbohydrates 24g

- Protein 3g

- Sodium 518mg

Baked Ginger Oatmeal with Pear Topping

Preparation Time: 10 minutes

Cooking Time: 15 minutes

Servings: 2

Difficulty Level: Easy

Ingredients:

- 1 cup of old-fashioned oats

- 3/4 cup of milk, fat-free (skim)

- 1 egg white

- 1 1/2 teaspoons of grated ginger, fresh or 3/4 teaspoon of ground ginger

- 2 tablespoons of brown sugar, divided

- 1/2 ripe diced pear

Directions:

1. Spray 2x6 ounce ramekins with a non-stick cooking spray. Prepare the oven to 350 ° F. Combine the first four ingredients and a tablespoon of sugar, then mix well. Pour evenly between the 2 ramekins. Top with pear slices and the remaining tablespoon of sugar. Bake for 15 minutes. Serve warm.

Nutrition (for 100g):

- Calories 268

- Fat 5g

- Carbohydrates 2g

- Protein 10g

- Sodium 779mg

Greek-Style Veggie Omelet

Preparation Time: 10 minutes

Cooking Time: 20 minutes

Servings: 2

Difficulty Level: Easy

Ingredients:

- 4 large eggs

- 2 tablespoons of fat-free milk

- 1/8 teaspoon of salt

- 3 teaspoons of olive oil, divided

- 2 cups of baby Portobello, sliced

- 1/4 cup of finely chopped onion

- 1 cup of fresh baby spinach

- 3 tablespoons of feta cheese, crumbled

- 2 tablespoons of ripe olives, sliced

- Freshly ground pepper

Directions:

1. Whisk together the first three ingredients. Stir in 2 tablespoons of oil in a non-stick skillet over medium-high heat. Sauté the onions and mushroom for 5-6 minutes or until golden brown. Mix in the spinach and cook. Remove mixture from pan.

2. Using the same pan, heat over medium-low heat the remaining oil. Pour your egg mixture and as it starts to set, pushed the edges towards the center to let the uncooked mixture flow underneath. When eggs are set, scoop the veggie mixture on one side. Sprinkle with olives and feta, then fold the other side to close. Slice in half and sprinkle with pepper to serve.

Nutrition (for 100g):

- Calories 271

- Fat 2g

- Carbohydrates 7g

- Protein 18g

- Sodium 648mg

Sweet Potatoes with Coconut Flakes

Preparation Time: 15 mins

Cooking Time: 1 hour

Servings: 2

Ingredients:

- 16 oz.. of sweet potatoes

- 1 tbsp. of maple syrup

- ¼ c. of Fat-free coconut Greek yogurt

- 1/8 c. of unsweetened toasted coconut flakes

- 1 chopped apple

Directions:

1. Preheat oven to 400 °F.

2. Place your potatoes on a baking sheet. Bake them for 45 - 60 minutes or until soft.

3. Use a sharp knife to mark "X" on the potatoes and fluff pulp with a fork.

4. Top with coconut flakes, chopped apple, Greek yogurt, and maple syrup.

5. Serve immediately.

Nutrition:

- Calories: 321

- Fat: 3 g

- Carbs: 70 g

- Protein: 7 g

- Sugars: 0.1 g

- Sodium: 3%

Flaxseed & Banana Smoothie

Preparation Time: 5 mins

Cooking Time: 0 mins

Servings: 1

Ingredients:

- 1 frozen banana

- ½ c. of almond milk

- Vanilla extract.

- 1 tbsp. of almond butter

- 2 tbsps. of Flax seed 1 tsp. maple syrup

Directions:

1. Add all your ingredients to a food processor or blender and run until smooth. Pour the mixture into a glass and enjoy.

Nutrition:

- Calories: 376

- Fat: 19.4 g

- Carbs: 48.3 g

- Protein: 9.2 g

- Sugars: 12%

- Sodium: 64.9 mg

Fruity Tofu Smoothie

Preparation Time: 5 mins

Cooking Time: 0 mins

Servings: 2

Ingredients:

- 1 c. of ice cold water

- 1 c. of packed spinach

- ¼ c. of frozen mango chunks

- ½ c. of frozen pineapple chunks

- 1 tbsp. of chia seeds

- 1 container of silken tofu

- 1 frozen medium banana

Directions:

1. In a powerful blender, add all ingredients and puree until smooth and creamy.

2. Evenly divide into two glasses, serve and enjoy.

Nutrition:

- Calories: 175

- Fat: 3.7 g

- Carbs: 33.3 g

- Protein: 6.0 g

- Sugars: 16.3 g

- Sodium: 1%

French Toast with Applesauce

Preparation Time: 5 mins

Cooking Time: 5 mins

Servings: 6

Ingredients:

- ¼ c. of unsweetened applesauce

- ½ c. of skim milk

- 2 packets of Stevia

- 2 eggs

- 6 slices of whole-wheat bread

- 1 tsp. of ground cinnamon

Directions:

1. Mix well applesauce, sugar, cinnamon, milk, and eggs in a mixing bowl.

2. One slice at a time, soak the bread into an applesauce mixture until wet.

3. On medium fire, heat a large nonstick skillet.

4. Add soaked bread on one side and another on the other side. Cook in a single layer in batches for 2-3 minutes per side on medium-low fire or until lightly browned.

5. Serve and enjoy.

Nutrition:

- Calories: 122.6

- Fat: 2.6 g

- Carbs: 18.3 g

- Protein: 6.5 g

- Sugars: 14.8 g

- Sodium: 11%

Banana-Peanut Butter 'n Greens Smoothie

Preparation Time: 5 mins

Cooking Time: 0 mins

Servings: 1

Ingredients:

- 1 c. of chopped and packed Romaine lettuce

- 1 frozen medium banana

- 1 tbsp. of all-natural peanut butter

- 1 c. of cold almond milk

Directions:

1. In a heavy-duty blender, add all ingredients.

2. Puree until smooth and creamy.

3. Serve and enjoy.

Nutrition:

- Calories: 349.3

- Fat: 9.7 g

- Carbs: 57.4 g

- Protein: 8.1 g

- Sugars: 4.3 g

- Sodium: 18%

Baking Powder Biscuits

Preparation Time: 5 mins

Cooking Time: 5 mins

Servings: 1

Ingredients:

- 1 egg white
- 1 c. of white whole-wheat flour
- 4 tbsps. of Non-hydrogenated vegetable shortening
- 1 tbsp. of sugar
- 2/3 c. of low-fat milk
- 1 c. of unbleached all-purpose flour
- 4 tsps. of Sodium-free baking powder

Directions:

1. Preheat oven to 450°F. Take out a baking sheet and set it aside.

2. Place the flour, sugar, and baking powder into a mixing bowl and whisk well to combine.

3. Cut the shortening into the mixture using your fingers, and work until it resembles coarse crumbs. Add the egg white and milk and stir to combine.

4. Turn the dough out onto a lightly floured surface and knead for 1 minute. Roll dough to ¾ inch thickness and cut into 12 rounds.

5. Place rounds on the baking sheet. Place baking sheet on middle rack in the oven and bake 10 minutes.

6. Remove baking sheet and place biscuits on a wire rack to cool.

Nutrition:

- Calories: 118

- Fat: 4 g

- Carbs: 16 g

- Protein: 3 g

- Sugars: 0.2 g

- Sodium: 6%

Oatmeal Banana Pancakes with Walnuts

Preparation Time: 15 mins

Cooking Time: 5 mins

Servings: 8 pancakes

Ingredients:

- 1 finely diced firm banana

- 1 c. of whole wheat pancake mix

- 1/8 c. of chopped walnuts

- ¼ c. of old-fashioned oats

Directions:

1. Make the pancake mix according to the directions on the package.

2. Add walnuts, oats, and chopped banana.

3. Coat a griddle with cooking spray. Add about ¼ cup of the pancake batter onto the griddle when hot.

4. Turn pancake over when bubbles form on top. Cook until golden brown.

5. Serve immediately.

Nutrition:

- Calories: 155

- Fat: 4 g

- Carbs: 28 g

- Protein: 7 g

- Sugars: 2.2 g

- Sodium: 16%

Creamy Oats, Greens & Blueberry Smoothie

Preparation Time: 4 mins

Cooking Time: 0 mins

Servings: 1

Ingredients:

- 1 c. of cold Fat-free milk

- 1 c. of salad greens

- ½ c. of fresh frozen blueberries

- ½ c. of frozen cooked oatmeal

- 1 tbsp. of sunflower seeds

Directions:

1. In a powerful blender, blend all ingredients until smooth and creamy.

2. Serve and enjoy.

Nutrition:

- Calories: 280

- Fat: 6.8 g

- Carbs: 44.0 g

- Protein: 14.0 g

- Sugars: 32 g

- Sodium: 141%

Banana & Cinnamon Oatmeal

Preparation Time: 5 mins

Cooking Time: 0 mins

Servings: 6

Ingredients:

- 2 c. of quick-cooking oats

- 4 c. of Fat-free milk

- 1 tsp. of ground cinnamon

- 2 chopped large ripe banana

- 4 tsps. of Brown sugar

- Extra ground cinnamon

Directions:

1. Place milk in a skillet and bring to boil. Add oats and cook over medium heat until thickened, for two to four minutes. Stir intermittently.

2. Add cinnamon, brown sugar, banana, and stir to combine.

3. If you want, serve with the extra cinnamon and milk. Enjoy!

Nutrition:

- Calories: 215

- Fat: 2 g

- Carbs: 42 g

- Protein: 10 g

- Sugars: 1 g

- Sodium: 40%

Bagels Made Healthy

Preparation Time: 5 mins

Cooking Time: 40 mins

Servings: 8

Ingredients:

- 1 ½ c. of warm water
- 1 ¼ c. of bread flour
- 2 tbsps. of Honey
- 2 c. of whole wheat flour
- 2 tsps. of Yeast
- 1 ½ tbsps. of Olive oil
- 1 tbsp. of vinegar

Directions:

1. In a bread machine, mix all ingredients, and then process on dough cycle.

2. Once done, create 8 pieces shaped like a flattened ball.

3. Make a hole in the center of each ball using your thumb then create a donut shape.

4. In a greased baking sheet, place donut-shaped dough then covers and let it rise about ½ hour.

5. Prepare about 2 inches of water to boil in a large pan.

6. In a boiling water, drop one at a time the bagels and boil for 1 minute, then turn them once.

7. Remove them and return to a baking sheet and bake at 350oF for about 20 to 25 minutes until golden brown.

Nutrition:

- Calories: 228.1; Fat: 3.7 g; Carbs: 41.8 g; Protein: 6.9 g; Sugars: 0 g ; Sodium: 15%

Chapter 4. Lunch Recipes

Kushari

Preparation Time: 25 minutes

Cooking Time: 1 hour and 20 minutes

Servings: 8

Difficulty Level: Difficult

Ingredients:

For the sauce:
- 2 tablespoons of olive oil

- 2 garlic cloves, minced

- 1 (16-ounce) can of tomato sauce

- ¼ cup of white vinegar

- ¼ cup of Harissa, or store-bought

- 1/8 teaspoon of salt

For the rice:
- 1 cup of olive oil

- 2 onions, thinly sliced

- 2 cups of dried brown lentils

- 4 quarts plus ½ cup of water, divided

- 2 cups of short-grain rice

- 1 teaspoon of salt

- 1-pound of short elbow pasta

- 1 (15-ounce) can of chickpeas, drained and rinsed

Directions:

To make the sauce:

1. In a saucepan, cook the olive oil. Sauté the garlic. Stir in the tomato sauce, vinegar, harissa, and salt. Bring the sauce to a boil. Turn down the heat to low and cook for 20 minutes or until the sauce has thickened. Remove and set aside.

To make the rice

1. Ready the plate with paper towels and set aside. In a large pan over medium heat, heat the olive oil. Sauté the onions, often stir, until crisp and golden. Transfer the onions to the prepared plate and set them aside. Reserve 2 tablespoons of the cooking oil. Reserve the pan.

2. Over high heat, combine the lentils and 4 cups of water in a pot. Allow it to boil and cook for 20 minutes. Strain and toss with the reserved 2 tablespoons of cooking oil. Set aside. Reserve the pot.

3. Place the pan you used to fry the onions over medium-high heat and add the rice, 4½ cups of water, and salt. Bring to a boil. Set the heat to low, and cook for 20 minutes. Turn off and set aside for 10 minutes. Bring the remaining 8 cups of water, salted, to a boil over high heat in the same pot used to cook the lentils. Drop

in the pasta and cook for 6 minutes or according to the package instructions. Drain and set aside.

<u>To assemble:</u>

1. Spoon the rice onto a serving platter. Top it with lentils, chickpeas, and pasta. Drizzle with the hot tomato sauce and sprinkle with the crispy fried onions.

Nutrition (for 100g):

- Calories668

- Fat 13g

- Carbohydrates 113g

- Protein 18g

- Sodium 481mg

Bulgur with Tomatoes and Chickpeas

Preparation Time: 10 minutes

Cooking Time: 35 minutes

Servings: 6

Difficulty Level: Average

Ingredients:

- ½ cup of olive oil

- 1 onion, chopped

- 6 tomatoes, diced, or 1 (16-ounce) can diced tomatoes

- 2 tablespoons of tomato paste

- 2 cups of water

- 1 tablespoon of Harissa, or store-bought

- 1/8 teaspoon of salt

- 2 cups of coarse bulgur

- 1 (15-ounce) can of chickpeas, drained and rinsed

Directions:

1. In a heavy-bottomed pot over medium heat, heat the olive oil. Sauté the onion, then add the tomatoes with their juice and cook for 5 minutes.

2. Stir in the tomato paste, water, harissa, and salt. Bring to a boil.

3. Stir in the bulgur and chickpeas. Return the mixture to a boil. Decrease the heat to low and cook for 15 minutes. Let rest for 15 minutes before serving.

Nutrition (for 100g):

- Calories 413

- Fat 19g

- Carbohydrates 55g

- Protein 14g

- Sodium 728mg

Mackerel Maccheroni

Preparation Time: 10 minutes

Cooking Time: 15 minutes

Servings: 4

Difficulty Level: Easy

Ingredients:

- 12 oz. of Maccheroni

- 1 clove garlic

- 14 oz. of Tomato sauce

- 1 sprig chopped parsley

- 2 Fresh chili peppers

- 1 teaspoon of salt

- 7 oz. of mackerel in oil

- 3 tablespoons of extra virgin olive oil

Directions:

1. Start by putting the water to a boil in a saucepan. While the water is heating up, take a pan, pour in a little oil and a little garlic, and cook over low heat. Once the garlic is cooked, pull it out from the pan.

2. Cut open the chili pepper, remove the internal seeds and cut into thin strips.

3. Add the cooking water and the chili pepper to the same pan as before. Then, take the mackerel, and after draining the oil and separating it with a fork, put it in the pan with the other ingredients. Lightly sauté it by adding some cooking water.

4. When all the ingredients are well incorporated, add the tomato puree to the pan. Mix well to even out all the ingredients and cook on low heat for about 3 minutes.

Let's move on to the pasta:

1. After the water starts boiling, add the salt and the pasta. Drain the maccheroni once they are slightly al dente, and add them to the sauce you prepared.

2. Sauté for a few moments in the sauce and after tasting, season with salt and pepper according to your liking.

Nutrition (for 100g):

- Calories 510

- Fat 15.4g

- Carbohydrates 70g

- Protein 22.9g

- Sodium 730mg

Maccheroni with Cherry Tomatoes and Anchovies

Preparation Time: 10 minutes

Cooking Time: 15 minutes

Servings: 4

Difficulty Level: Easy

Ingredients:

- 14 oz. of Maccheroni Pasta

- 6 Salted anchovies

- 4 oz. of Cherry tomatoes

- 1 clove garlic

- 3 tablespoons of extra virgin olive oil

- Fresh chili peppers to taste

- 3 basil leaves

- Salt to taste

Directions:

1. Start by heating water in a pot and add salt when it is boiling. Meanwhile, prepare the sauce: take the tomatoes after having washed them and cut them into 4 pieces.

2. Now, take a non-stick pan, sprinkle in a little oil, and throw in a clove of garlic. Once cooked, remove it from the pan. Add the clean anchovies to the pan, melting them in the oil.

3. When the anchovies are well dissolved, add the cut tomatoes pieces and turn the heat up to high until they begin to soften (be careful not to let them become too soft).

4. Add the chili peppers without seeds, cut into small pieces, and season.

5. Transfer the pasta to the pot of boiling water, drain it al dente, and let it sauté in the saucepan for a few moments.

Nutrition (for 100g):

- Calories 476

- Fat 11g

- Carbohydrates 81.4g

- Protein 12.9g

- Sodium 763mg

Lemon and Shrimp Risotto

Preparation Time: 10 minutes

Cooking Time: 30 minutes

Servings: 4

Difficulty Level: Easy

Ingredients:

- 1 lemon

- 14 oz. of Shelled shrimp

- 1 ¾ cups of risotto rice

- 1 white onion

- 33 fl. oz. (1 liter) of vegetable broth (even less is fine)

- 2 ½ tablespoons of butter

- ½ glass of white wine

- Salt to taste

- Black pepper to taste

- Chives to taste

Directions:

1. Start by boiling the shrimps in salted water for 3-4 minutes, drain and set aside.

2. Peel and finely chop an onion, stir-fry it with melted butter and once the butter has dried, toast the rice in the pan for a few minutes.

3. Deglaze the rice with half a glass of white wine, then add the juice of 1 lemon. Stir and finish cooking the rice by continuing to add a spoon of vegetable stock as needed.

4. Mix well and a few minutes before the end of cooking, add the previously cooked shrimps (keeping some of them aside for garnish) and some black pepper.

5. Once the heat is off, add a knob of butter and stir. The risotto is ready to be served. Decorate with the remaining shrimp and sprinkle with some chives.

Nutrition (for 100g):

- Calories 510

- Fat 10g

- Carbohydrates 82.4g

- Protein 20.6g

1. Sodium 875mg

Spaghetti with Clams

Preparation Time: 10 minutes

Cooking Time: 40 minutes

Servings: 4

Difficulty Level: Easy

Ingredients:

- 11.5 oz. of spaghetti

- 2 pounds of clams

- 7 oz. of tomato sauce, or tomato pulp, for the red version of this dish

- 2 cloves of garlic

- 4 tablespoons of extra virgin olive oil

- 1 glass of dry white wine

- 1 tablespoon of finely chopped parsley

- 1 chili pepper

Directions:

1. Start by washing the clams: never "purge" the clams—they must only be opened through the use of heat; otherwise, their precious internal liquid is lost along with any sand. Wash the clams quickly using a colander placed in a salad bowl: this will filter out the sand on the shells.

2. Then immediately put the drained clams in a saucepan with a lid on high heat. Turn them over occasionally, and when they are almost all open, take them off the heat. The clams that remain closed are dead and must be eliminated. Remove the mollusks from the open ones, leaving some of them whole to decorate the dishes. Strain the liquid left at the bottom of the pan, and set it aside.

3. Take a large pan and pour a little oil into it. Heat a whole pepper and one or two cloves of crushed garlic on very low heat until the cloves become yellowish. Add the clams and season with dry white wine.

4. Now, add the clam liquid strained previously and some finely chopped parsley.

5. Strain and immediately toss the spaghetti al dente in the pan after having cooked them in plenty of salted water. Stir well until the spaghetti absorbs all the liquid from the clams. If you did not use a chili pepper, complete with a light sprinkle of white or black pepper.

Nutrition (for 100g):

- Calories 167

- Fat 8g

- Carbohydrates 8.63g

- Protein 5g

- Sodium 720mg

Greek Fish Soup

Preparation Time: 10 minutes

Cooking Time: 60 minutes

Servings: 4

Difficulty Level: Easy

Ingredients:

- Hake or other white fish

- 4 Potatoes

- 4 Spring onions

- 2 Carrots

- 2 stalks of Celery

- 2 Tomatoes

- 4 tablespoons of Extra virgin olive oil

- 2 Eggs

- 1 Lemon

- 1 cup of Rice

- Salt to taste

Directions:

1. Choose a fish not exceeding 2.2pounds in weight, remove its scales, gills, and intestines and wash it well. Salt it and set it aside.

2. Wash the potatoes, carrots, and onions and put them in the saucepan whole with enough water to soak them and then bring to a boil.

3. Add in the celery still tied in bunches, so it does not disperse while cooking; cut the tomatoes into four parts and add these too, together with oil and salt.

4. When the vegetables are almost cooked, add more water and the fish. Boil for 20 minutes, then remove it from the broth together with the vegetables.

5. Place the fish in a serving dish by adorning it with the vegetables and strain the broth. Put the broth back on the heat, diluting it with a little water. Once it boils, put in the rice and season with salt. Once the rice is cooked, remove the saucepan from the heat.

Prepare the avgolemono sauce:

1. Beat the eggs well and slowly add the lemon juice. Put some broth in a ladle and slowly pour it into the eggs, mixing constantly.

2. Finally, add the obtained sauce to the soup and mix well.

Nutrition (for 100g):

- Calories 263

- Fat 17.1g

- Carbohydrates 18.6g

- Protein 9g

- Sodium 823mg

Venere Rice with Shrimp

Preparation Time: 10 minutes

Cooking Time: 55 minutes

Servings: 3

Difficulty Level: Easy

Ingredients:

- 1 ½ cups of black Venere rice (better if parboiled)

- 5 teaspoons of extra virgin olive oil

- 10.5 oz. of shrimp

- 10.5 oz. of zucchini

- 1 Lemon (juice and rind)

- Table Salt to taste

- Black pepper to taste

- 1 clove garlic

- Tabasco to taste

Directions:

Let's start with the rice:

1. After filling a pot with plenty of water and bringing it to a boil, pour in the rice, add salt, and cook for the necessary time (check the package's cooking instructions).

2. Meanwhile, grate the zucchini with a grater with large holes. In a pan, heat the olive oil with the peeled garlic clove, add the grated zucchini, salt, and pepper, cook for 5 minutes; remove the garlic clove, and set the vegetables aside.

Now clean the shrimp:

1. Remove the shell, cut the tail, divide them in half lengthwise, and remove the intestine (the dark thread in their back). Situate the cleaned shrimps in a bowl and season with olive oil; give it some

extra flavor by adding lemon zest, salt, and pepper and by adding a few drops of Tabasco if you so choose.

2. Heat up the shrimps in a hot pan for a couple of minutes. Once cooked, set aside.

3. Once the Venere rice is ready, strain it in a bowl, add the zucchini mix, and stir.

Nutrition (for 100g):

- Calories 293

- Fat 5g

- Carbohydrates 52g

- Protein 10g

- Sodium 655mg

Pennette with Salmon and Vodka

Preparation Time: 10 minutes

Cooking Time: 18 minutes

Servings: 4

Difficulty Level: Easy

Ingredients:

- 14 oz. of Pennette Rigate

- 7 oz. of Smoked salmon

- 1.2 oz. of Shallot

- 1.35 fl. oz..(40ml) of Vodka

- 5 oz.. of cherry tomatoes

- 7 oz.. of fresh liquid cream (I recommend the vegetable one for a lighter dish)

- Chives to taste

- 3 tablespoons of extra virgin olive oil

- Salt to taste

- Black pepper to taste

- Basil to taste (for garnish)

Directions:

1. Wash and cut the tomatoes and the chives. After having peeled the shallot, chop it with a knife, put it in a saucepan, and let it marinate in extra virgin olive oil for a few moments.

2. Meanwhile, cut the salmon into strips and sauté it together with the oil and shallot.

3. Blend everything with the vodka, being careful as there could be a flare (if a flame should rise, don't worry, it will lower as soon as

the alcohol has evaporated completely). Add the chopped tomatoes and add a pinch of salt and, if you like, some pepper. Finally, add the cream and chopped chives.

4. While the sauce continues cooking, prepare the pasta. Once the water boils, pour in the Pennette and let them cook until al dente.

5. Strain the pasta, and pour the Pennette into the sauce, letting them cook for a few moments so as allow them to absorb all the flavor. If you like, garnish with a basil leaf.

Nutrition (for 100g):

- Calories 620

- Fat 21.9g

- Carbohydrates81.7g

- Protein 24g

- Sodium 326mg

Seafood Carbonara

Preparation Time: 15 minutes

Cooking Time: 50 minutes

Servings: 3

Difficulty Level: Easy

Ingredients:

- 11.5 oz. of Spaghetti

- 3.5 oz. of Tuna

- 3.5 oz. of Swordfish

- 3.5 oz. of Salmon

- 6 Yolks

- 4 tablespoons of Parmesan cheese (Parmigiano Reggiano)

- 2 fl. oz.. (60ml) of White wine

- 1 clove garlic

- Extra virgin olive oil to taste

- Table Salt to taste

- Black pepper to taste

Directions:

1. Prepare a boiling water in a pot and add a little salt.

2. Meanwhile, pour 6 egg yolks in a bowl and add the grated parmesan, pepper, and salt. Beat with a whisk, and dilute with a little cooking water from the pot.

3. Remove any bones from the salmon, the scales from the swordfish, and proceed by dicing the tuna, salmon, and swordfish.

4. Once it boils, toss in the pasta and cook it slightly al dente.

5. Meanwhile, heat a little oil in a large pan, add the whole peeled garlic clove. Once the oil is hot, toss in the fish cubes and sauté over high heat for about 1 minute. Remove the garlic and add the white wine.

6. Once the alcohol evaporates, take out the fish cubes and lower the heat. As soon as the spaghetti is ready, add them to the pan and sauté for about a minute, stirring constantly and adding the cooking water, as needed.

7. Pour in the egg yolk mixture and the fish cubes. Mix well. Serve.

Nutrition (for 100g):

- Calories 375

- Fat 17g

- Carbohydrates 41.40g

- Protein 14g

- Sodium 755 mg

Garganelli with Zucchini Pesto and Shrimp

Preparation Time: 10 minutes

Cooking Time: 30 minutes

Servings: 4

Difficulty Level: Average

Ingredients:

- 14 oz. egg-based Garganelli

- For the zucchini pesto:

- 7oz. Zucchini

- 1 cup Pine nuts

- 8 tablespoons (0.35oz.) Basil

- 1 teaspoon of table salt

- 9 tablespoons extra virgin olive oil

- 2 tablespoons Parmesan cheese to be grated

- 1oz. of Pecorino to be grated

- For the sautéed shrimp:

- 8.8oz. shrimp

- 1 clove garlic

- 7 teaspoons extra virgin olive oil

- Pinch of Salt

Directions:

Start by preparing the pesto:

1. After washing the zucchini, grate them, place them in a colander (to allow them to lose some excess liquid), and lightly salt them. Put the pine nuts, zucchini and basil leaves in the blender. Add the grated Parmesan, the pecorino, and the extra virgin olive oil.

2. Blend everything until the mixture is creamy, stir in a pinch of salt, and set aside.

Switch to the shrimp:

1. First of all, pull out the intestine by cutting the shrimp's back with a knife along its entire length and, with the tip of the knife, remove the black thread inside.

2. Cook the clove of garlic in a non-stick pan with extra virgin olive oil. When it's browned, remove the garlic and add the shrimps. Sauté them for about 5 minutes over medium heat until you see a crispy crust form on the outside.

3. Then, boil a pot of salted water and cook the Garganelli. Set a couple of spoons of cooking water aside, and drain the pasta al dente.

4. Put the Garganelli in the pan where you cooked the shrimp. Cook together for a minute, add a spoon of cooking water and finally, add the zucchini pesto.

5. Mix everything well to combine the pasta with the sauce.

Nutrition (for 100g):

- Calories 776

- Fat 46g

- Carbohydrates 68g

- Protein 22.5g

- Sodium 835mg

Salmon Risotto

Preparation Time: 10 minutes

Cooking Time: 30 minutes

Servings: 4

Difficulty Level: Average

Ingredients:

- 1 ¾ cup (12.3 oz..) of Rice

- 8.8 oz. of Salmon steaks

- 1 Leek

- Extra virgin olive oil to taste

- 1 clove of garlic

- ½ glass of white wine

- 3 ½ tablespoons of grated Grana Padano

- salt to taste

- Black pepper to taste

- 17 fl. oz. (500ml) of Fish broth

- 1 cup of butter

Directions:

1. Start by cleaning the salmon and cutting it into small pieces. Cook 1 tablespoon of oil in a pan with a whole garlic clove and brown the salmon for 2/3 minutes, add salt, and set the salmon aside, removing the garlic.

Now, start preparing the risotto:

1. Cut the leek into very small pieces and let it simmer in a pan over low heat with two oil tablespoons. Stir in the rice and cook it for a few seconds over medium-high heat, stirring with a wooden spoon.

2. Stir in the white wine, continue cooking, stir occasionally, try not to let the rice stick to the pan, and gradually add the stock (vegetable or fish).

3. Halfway through cooking, add the salmon, butter, and a pinch of salt if necessary. When the rice is well cooked, remove it from heat. Combine with a couple of tablespoons of grated Grana Padano and serve.

Nutrition (for 100g):

- Calories 521

- Fat 13g

- Carbohydrates 82g

- Protein 19g

- Sodium 839mg

Chapter 5.   Dinner Recipes

Stuffed Bell Peppers

Preparation Time: 10 minutes

Cooking Time: 25 minutes

Servings: 4

Ingredients:

- 4 bell peppers

- 1 ½ cup of ground beef 1 zucchini, grated

- 1 white onion, diced

- ½ teaspoon of ground nutmeg

- 1 tablespoon of olive oil

- 1 teaspoon of ground black pepper

- ½ teaspoon of salt

- 3 oz. Parmesan, grated

Directions:

1. Cut the bell peppers into halves and remove seeds.

2. Place ground beef in the skillet.

3. Add grated zucchini, diced onion, ground nutmeg, olive oil, ground black pepper, and salt.

4. Roast the mixture for 5 minutes.

5. Place bell pepper halves in the tray.

6. Fill every pepper half with ground beef mixture and top with grated Parmesan.

7. Cover the tray with foil and secure the edges.

8. Cook the stuffed bell peppers for 20 minutes at 360°F.

Nutrition:

- Calories 241

- Fat 14.6

- Fiber 3.4

- Carbs 11

- Protein 18.6

- Sodium 37%

Stuffed Eggplants with Goat Cheese

Preparation Time: 15 minutes

Cooking Time: 25 minutes

Servings: 4

Ingredients:

- 1 large eggplant, trimmed

- 1 tomato, crushed

- 1 garlic clove, diced

- ½ teaspoon of ground black pepper

- ½ teaspoon of smoked paprika

- 1 cup of spinach, chopped

- 4 oz.. of goat cheese, crumbled

- 1 teaspoon of butter

- 2 oz.. of Cheddar cheese, shredded

Directions:

1. Cut the eggplants into halves and then cut every half into 2 parts.

2. Remove the flesh from the eggplants to get eggplant boards.

3. Mix up together crushed tomato, diced garlic, ground black pepper, smoked paprika, chopped spinach, crumbled goat cheese, and butter.

4. Fill the eggplants with this mixture.

5. Top every eggplant board with shredded Cheddar cheese.

6. Put the eggplants in the tray.

7. Preheat the oven to 365 °F.

8. Place the tray with eggplants in the oven and cook for 25 minutes.

Nutrition:

- Calories 229

- Fat 16.1

- Fiber 4.6

- Carbs 9

- Protein 13.8

- Sodium 21%

Korma Curry

Preparation Time: 10 minutes

Cooking Time: 25 minutes

Servings: 6

Ingredients:

- 3-pound of chicken breast, skinless, boneless

- 1 teaspoon of garam masala

- 1 teaspoon of curry powder

- 1 tablespoon of apple cider vinegar

- ½ teaspoon of coconut cream

- 1 cup of organic almond milk

- 1 teaspoon of ground coriander

- ¾ teaspoon of ground cardamom

- ½ teaspoon of ginger powder

- ¼ teaspoon of cayenne pepper

- ¾ teaspoon of ground cinnamon

- 1 tomato, diced 1 teaspoon avocado oil

- ½ cup of water

Directions:

1. Chop the chicken breast and put it in the saucepan.

2. Add avocado oil and start to cook it over medium heat.

3. Sprinkle the chicken with garam masala, curry powder, apple cider vinegar, ground coriander, cardamom, ginger powder, cayenne pepper, ground cinnamon, and diced tomato. Mix up the ingredients carefully. Cook them for 10 minutes.

4. Add water, coconut cream, and almond milk. Sauté the meat for 10 minutes more.

Nutrition:

- Calories 411

- Fat 19.3

- Fiber 0.9

- Carbs 6

- Protein 49.9

- Sodium 12%

Zucchini Bars

Preparation Time: 10 minutes

Cooking Time: 15 minutes

Servings: 8

Ingredients:

- 3 zucchinis, grated

- ½ white onion, diced

- 2 teaspoons of butter

- 3 eggs, whisked

- 4 tablespoons of coconut flour

- 1 teaspoon of salt

- ½ teaspoon of ground black pepper

- 5 oz.. of goat cheese, crumbled

- ½ cup of spinach, chopped

- 1 teaspoon of baking powder

- ½ teaspoon of lemon juice

Directions:

1. In the mixing bowl, mix up together grated zucchini, diced onion, eggs, coconut flour, salt, ground black pepper, crumbled cheese, chopped spinach, baking powder, and lemon juice.

2. Add butter and churn the mixture until homogenous.

3. Line the baking dish with baking paper.

4. Transfer the zucchini mixture to the baking dish and flatten it.

5. Preheat the oven to 365°F and put the dish inside.

6. Cook it for 15 minutes. Then chill the meal well.

7. Cut it into bars.

Nutrition:

- Calories 199

- Fat 1316

- Fiber 215

- Carbs 7.1

- Protein 13.1

- Sodium 21%

Mushroom Soup

Preparation Time: 10 minutes

Cooking Time: 25 minutes

Servings: 4

Ingredients:

- 1 cup of water

- 1 cup of coconut milk

- 1 cup of white mushrooms, chopped

- ½ carrot, chopped

- ¼ white onion, diced

- 1 tablespoon of butter

- 2 oz.. of turnip, chopped

- 1 teaspoon of dried dill

- ½ teaspoon of ground black pepper

- ¾ teaspoon of smoked paprika

- 1 oz.. of celery stalk, chopped

Directions:

1. Pour water and coconut milk into the saucepan. Bring the liquid to a boil. Add chopped mushrooms, carrots, and turnips. Close the lid and boil for 10 minutes.

2. Meanwhile, put butter in the skillet. Add diced onion. Sprinkle it with dill, ground black pepper, and smoked paprika. Roast the onion for 3 minutes. Add the roasted onion to the soup mixture.

3. Then add chopped celery stalk. Close the lid.

4. Cook soup for 10 minutes.

5. Then ladle it into the serving bowls.

Nutrition:

- Calories 181

- Fat 17.3

- Fiber 2.5

- Carbs 6.9

- Protein 2.4

- Sodium 4%

Stuffed Portobello Mushrooms

Preparation Time: 10 minutes

Cooking Time: 10 minutes

Servings: 4

Ingredients:

- 2 Portobello mushrooms

- 2 oz.. of artichoke hearts, drained, chopped

- 1 tablespoon of coconut cream

- 1 tablespoon of cream cheese

- 1 teaspoon of minced garlic

- 1 tablespoon of fresh cilantro, chopped

- 3 oz.. of Cheddar cheese, grated

- ½ teaspoon of ground black pepper

- 2 tablespoons of olive oil

- ½ teaspoon of salt

Directions:

1. Sprinkle mushrooms with olive oil and place them in the tray. Transfer the tray in the preheated oven to 360 °F and broil them for 5 minutes.

2. Meanwhile, blend together artichoke hearts, coconut cream, cream cheese, minced garlic, and chopped cilantro. Add grated cheese in the mixture and sprinkle with ground black pepper and

salt. Fill the broiled mushrooms with the cheese mixture and cook them for 5 minutes more. Serve the mushrooms only hot.

Nutrition:

- Calories 183

- Fat 16.3

- Fiber 1.9

- Carbs 3

- Protein 7.7

- Sodium 37%

Lettuce Salad

Preparation Time: 10 minutes

Cooking Time: 0 minutes

Servings: 1

Ingredients:

- 1 cup of Romaine lettuce, roughly chopped

- 3 oz. of seitan, chopped

- 1 tablespoon of avocado oil

- 1 teaspoon of sunflower seeds

- 1 teaspoon of lemon juice

- 1 egg boiled, peeled

- 2 oz. of Cheddar cheese, shredded

Directions:

1. Place lettuce in the salad bowl. Add chopped seitan and Cheddar cheese.

2. Then chop the egg roughly and add it to the salad bowl too.

3. Mix up together lemon juice with the avocado oil.

4. Sprinkle the salad with the oil mixture and sunflower seeds. Don't stir the salad before serving.

Nutrition:

- Calories 663

- Fat 29.5

- Fiber 4.7

- Carbs 3.8

- Protein 84.2

- Sodium 45%

Lemon Garlic Salmon

Preparation Time: 3 minutes

Cooking Time: 17 minutes

Servings: 4

Ingredients:

- 2 pounds of salmon fillets, frozen

- 1 cup of water

- ¼ teaspoon of garlic powder

- 1/8 teaspoon of pepper

- ¼ cup of lemon juice

- ¼ teaspoon of salt to taste

- 1 lemon

Directions:

1. Put water into the instant pot and the lemon juice, then add the herbs and put it in a steamer rack.

2. Drizzle salmon with oil and season with pepper and salt.

3. Add garlic powder over salmon.

4. Layer the lemon slices over salmon.

5. Cook on manual high pressure for 7 minutes, then natural pressure release.

6. Enjoy over salad or some roasted veggies!

Nutrition:

- Calories: 165

- Fat: 10gg

- Carbs: 8g

- Net Carbs: 4g

- Protein: 15g

- Fiber: 4g

- Sodium 75%

Chickpea Curry

Preparation Time: 10 minutes

Cooking Time: 10 minutes

Servings: 6

Ingredients:

- 2 tablespoons of olive oil

- 1 diced small green pepper

- 2 cans of chickpeas, drained

- 1 cup of corn

- 1 cup of kale leaves

- 1 tablespoon of sugar-free maple syrup

- 1 diced onion

- 2 minced cloves of garlic

- 1 can of diced tomatoes with juice

- 1 cup of sliced okra

- 1 cup of vegetable broth

- 1 teaspoon of sea salt

- Juice of a lime

- ¼ teaspoon of ground black pepper

- 2 tablespoons of cilantro leaves

Directions:

1. Turn on the sauté function on the instant pot.

2. Cook onion for four minutes until browned, and then add in garlic and pepper and cook for 2 more minutes.

3. Add in curry powder and stir for 30 seconds, and then add the rest of the ingredients and seal the vent.

4. Cook under manual pressure for 5 minutes and then release natural pressure.

5. Add in the salt, pepper, and lime juice, and add more salt as needed.

6. Serve over cooked rice or top with cilantro leaves.

Nutrition:

- Calories: 119

- Fat: 5g

- Carbs: 18g

- Net Carbs: 16g

- Protein: 2g

- Fiber: 2g

- Sodium 30%

Instant Pot Chicken Thighs with Olives and Capers

Preparation Time: 15 minutes

Cooking Time: 20 minutes

Servings: 6

Ingredients:

- 6 chicken thighs

- 3 tablespoons of avocado oil

- ¼ teaspoon of sweet paprika

- A couple of small lemons

- 1 cup of chicken stock

- 1 cup of pitted olives

- 3 tablespoons of parsley leaves for garnish

- 1 teaspoon of kosher salt

- 1 teaspoon of ground turmeric

- ¼ teaspoon of black pepper

- ¼ teaspoon of mustard powder

- 2 tablespoons of cooking fat of choice

- 2 chopped cloves of garlic

- 2 tablespoons of capers

Directions:

1. Season chicken thighs with salt and put them in a baking dish.

2. Mix the spices with the avocado oil, put it over the chicken, put the marinate in there, and marinate for 20-30 minutes.

3. Halve the lemons, and then heat the ghee, swirling to the pot bottom. Brown the chickens for 3 minutes undisturbed, and then brown the second side.

4. Do this with the rest of the chicken, and then use the broth to deglaze the pot.

5. Put lemons at the bottom and chicken over the top, and then the rest of the ingredients over the chicken.

6. Let it cook for 14 minutes.

7. When finished, let natural pressure release, and then taste to see if it's ready, and put olives and capers over the chicken, garnishing with parsley.

Nutrition:

- Calories: 253

- Fat: 6g

- Carbs: 10gNet

- Carbs: 6g

- Protein: 13g

- Fiber: 4g

- Sodium 60%

Instant Pot salmon

Preparation Time: 5 minutes

Cooking Time: 15 minutes

Servings: 4

Ingredients:

- 1 cup of water

- 1 pound of salmon, cut into fillets

- Salt and pepper to taste

Directions:

1. Put a cup of water into the instant pot and add the trivet.

2. Put the fillets on top of that and add the salt and pepper onto it.

3. Secure and turn on the release valve to seal, and then cook on manual high pressure for 3 minutes or 5 minutes for frozen fillets.

4. When finished, let it vent and release the pressure, and serve with sauce or side dish.

Nutrition:

- Calories: 161

- Fat: 4g

- Carbs: 0

- Net Carbs: 0

- Protein: 22g

- Fiber: 0g

- Sodium 33%

Instant Pot Mac N' Cheese

Preparation Time: 10 minutes

Cooking Time: 10 minutes

Servings: 6

Ingredients:

- 1 cup of raw cashews, soaked
- ¼ cup of Nutritional yeast
- 1 tablespoon of apple cider vinegar
- 12 ounces of gluten-free pasta
- 5 cups of water, divided
- 2 teaspoons of sea salt
- 2 tablespoons of lemon juice
- 1//4 teaspoon of nutmeg

Directions:

1. Drain cashews and then combine them with 2 cups of water, yeast, lemon juice, vinegar, and nutmeg, and then blend until smooth.

2. Add pasta to the instant pot, put sauce on top, use two cups of water to rinse out the blender, pour water from the blender into the instant pot, and then seal and cook on manual pressure for 0 minutes, then let it natural pressure release.

3. Release steam and then put the rest of the water into a pot and use a spoon to stir.

4. Adjust seasonings, and you can add veggies and such to this.

Nutrition:

Calories: 329; Fat: 10g; Carbs: 52g; Net Carbs: 50g; Protein: 7g; Fiber: 2g
Sodium 84%

Chapter 6.   Dessert Recipes

The Most Elegant Parsley Soufflé Ever

Servings: 5

Preparation Time: 5 minutes

Cooking Time: 6 minutes

Ingredients:

2 whole eggs

1 fresh red chili pepper, chopped

2 tablespoons coconut cream

1 tablespoon fresh parsley, chopped

Sunflower seeds to taste

Directions:

Pre-heat your oven to 390 degrees F.

Almond butter 2 soufflé dishes.

Add the ingredients to a blender and mix well.

Divide batter into soufflé dishes and bake for 6 minutes.

Serve and enjoy!

Nutrition:

Calories: 108

Fat: 9g

Carbohydrates: 9g

Protein: 6g

Sodium 14%

Fennel and Almond Bites

Servings: 12

Preparation Time: 10 minutes

Cooking Time: None

Freeze Time:3 hours

Ingredients:

1 teaspoon vanilla extract

¼ cup almond milk

¼cup cocoa powder

½ cup almond oil

A pinch of sunflower seeds

1 teaspoon fennel seeds

Directions:

Take a bowl and mix the almond oil and almond milk.

Beat until smooth and glossy using electric beater.

Mix in the rest of the ingredients.

Take a piping bag and pour into a parchment paper lined baking sheet.

Freeze for 3 hours and store in the fridge.

Nutrition:

Total

Carbs: 1g

Fiber: 1g

Protein: 1g

Fat: 20g Sodium 3%

Feisty Coconut Fudge

Servings: 12

Preparation Time: 20 minutes

Cooking Time: None

Freeze Time: 2 hours

Ingredients:

¼ cup coconut, shredded

2 cups coconut oil

½ cup coconut cream

¼ cup almonds, chopped

1 teaspoon almond extract

A pinch of sunflower seeds

Stevia to taste

Directions:

Take a large bowl and pour coconut cream and coconut oil into it.

Whisk using an electric beater.

Whisk until the mixture becomes smooth and glossy.

Add cocoa powder slowly and mix well.

Add in the rest of the ingredients.

Pour into a bread pan lined with parchment paper.

Freeze until set.

Cut them into squares and serve.

Nutrition:

Total Carbs: 1g Fiber: 1g Protein: 0g

Fat: 20g Sodium 5%

No Bake Cheesecake

Servings: 10

Preparation Time: 120 minutes

Cooking Time: Nil

Ingredients: For Crust

2 tablespoons ground flaxseeds

2 tablespoons desiccated coconut

1 teaspoon cinnamon

For Filling

4 ounces' vegan cream cheese

1 cup cashews, soaked

½ cup frozen blueberries

2 tablespoons coconut oil

1 tablespoon lemon juice

1 teaspoon vanilla extract

Liquid stevia

Directions:

Take a container and mix in the crust ingredients, mix well.

Flatten the mixture at the bottom to prepare the crust of your cheesecake.

Take a blender/ food processor and add the filling ingredients, blend until smooth.

Gently pour the batter on top of your crust and chill for 2 hours. Serve and enjoy!

Nutrition:

Calories: 182 Fat: 16g Carbohydrates: 4g

Protein: 3g Sodium 36%

Easy Chia Seed Pumpkin Pudding

Servings: 4

Preparation Time: 10-15 minutes/ overnight chill time

Cooking Time: Nil

Ingredients:

1 cup maple syrup

2 teaspoons pumpkin spice

1 cup pumpkin puree

1 ¼ cup almond milk

½ cup chia seeds

Directions:

Add all of the ingredients to a bowl and gently stir.

Let it refrigerate overnight or at least 15 minutes.

Top with your desired ingredients, such as blueberries, almonds, etc.

Serve and enjoy!

Nutrition:

Calories: 230

Fat: 10g

Carbohydrates:22g

Protein:11g

Sodium 37%

Lovely Blueberry Pudding

Servings: 4

Preparation Time: 20 minutes

Cooking Time: Nil

Smart Points: 0

Ingredients:

2 cups frozen blueberries

2 teaspoons lime zest, grated freshly

20 drops liquid stevia

2 small avocados, peeled, pitted and chopped

½ teaspoon fresh ginger, grated freshly

4 tablespoons fresh lime juice

10 tablespoons water

Directions:

Add all of the listed ingredients to a blender (except blueberries) and pulse the mixture well.

Transfer the mix into small serving bowls and chill the bowls.

Serve with a topping of blueberries.

Enjoy!

Nutrition:

Calories: 166

Fat: 13g

Carbohydrates: 13g

Protein: 1.7g

Sodium 2%

Decisive Lime and Strawberry Popsicle

Servings: 4

Preparation Time: 2 hours

Cooking Time: Nil

Ingredients:

1 tablespoon lime juice, fresh

¼ cup strawberries, hulled and sliced

¼ cup coconut almond milk, unsweetened and full

Fat

2 teaspoons natural sweetener

Directions:

Blend the listed ingredients in a blender until smooth.

Pour mix into popsicle molds and let them chill for 2 hours.

Serve and enjoy!

Nutrition:

Calories: 166

Fat: 17g

Carbohydrates: 3g

Protein: 1g

Sodium 2%

Ravaging Blueberry Muffin

Servings: 4

Preparation Time: 10 minutes

Cooking Time: 30 minutes

Ingredients:

1 cup almond flour

Pinch of sunflower seeds

1/8 teaspoon baking soda

1 whole egg

2 tablespoons coconut oil, melted

½ cup coconut almond milk

¼ cup fresh blueberries

Directions:

Pre-heat your oven to 350 degrees F.

Line a muffin tin with paper muffin cups.

Add almond flour, sunflower seeds, baking soda to a bowl and mix, keep it on the side.

Take another bowl and add egg coconut oil, coconut almond milk and mix.

Add mix to flour mix and gently combine until incorporated.

Mix in blueberries and fill the cupcakes tins with batter.

Bake for 20-25 minutes.

Enjoy!

Nutrition:

Calories: 167 Fat: 15g Carbohydrates: 2.1g Protein: 5.2g Sodium 13%

The Coconut Loaf

Servings: 4

Preparation Time: 15 minutes

Cooking Time: 40 minutes

Ingredients:

1 ½ tablespoons coconut flour

¼ teaspoon baking powder

1/8 teaspoon sunflower seeds

1 tablespoons coconut oil, melted

1 whole egg

Directions:

Pre-heat your oven to 350 degrees F.

Add coconut flour, baking powder, sunflower seeds.

Add coconut oil, eggs and stir well until mixed.

Leave batter for several minutes.

Pour half batter onto baking pan.

Spread it to form a circle, repeat with remaining batter.

Bake in oven for 10 minutes.

Once you have a golden brown texture, let it cool and serve.

Enjoy!

Nutrition:

Calories: 297 Fat: 14g

Carbohydrates: 15g Protein: 15g

Sodium 8%

Fresh Figs with Walnuts and Ricotta

Servings: 4

Preparation Time: 5 minutes

Cooking Time: 2-3 minutes

Ingredients:

8 dried figs, halved

¼ cup ricotta cheese

16 walnuts, halved

1 tablespoon honey

Directions:

Take a skillet and place it over medium heat, add walnuts and toast for 2 minutes.

Top figs with cheese and walnuts.

Drizzle honey on top.

Enjoy!

Nutrition:

Calories: 142

Fat: 8g

Carbohydrates:10g

Protein:4g

Sodium 5%

Authentic Medjool Date Truffles

Servings: 4

Preparation Time: 10-15 minutes

Cooking Time: Nil

Ingredients:

2 tablespoons peanut oil

½ cup popcorn kernels

1/3 cup peanuts, chopped

1/3 cup peanut almond butter

¼ cup wildflower honey

Directions:

Take a pot and add popcorn kernels, peanut oil.

Place it over medium heat and shake the pot gently until all corn has popped.

Take a saucepan and add honey, gently simmer for 2-3 minutes.

Add peanut almond butter and stir.

Coat popcorn with the mixture and enjoy!

Nutrition:

Calories: 430

Fat: 20g

Carbohydrates: 56g

Protein 9g

Sodium 69%

Tasty Mediterranean Peanut Almond Butter Popcorns

Servings: 4

Preparation Time: 5 minutes + 20 minutes' chill time

Cooking Time: 2-3 minutes

Ingredients:

3 cups Medjool dates, chopped

12 ounces brewed coffee

1 cup pecans, chopped

½ cup coconut, shredded

½ cup cocoa powder

Directions:

Soak dates in warm coffee for 5 minutes.

Remove dates from coffee and mash them, making a fine smooth mixture.

Stir in remaining ingredients (except cocoa powder) and form small balls out of the mixture.

Coat with cocoa powder, serve and enjoy!

Nutrition:

Calories: 265

Fat: 12g

Carbohydrates: 43g

Protein 3g

Sodium 9%

Just A Minute Worth Muffin

Servings: 2

Preparation Time: 5 minutes

Cooking Time: 1 minute

Ingredients:

Coconut oil for grease

2 teaspoons coconut flour

1 pinch baking soda

1 pinch sunflower seeds

1 whole egg

Directions:

Grease ramekin dish with coconut oil and keep it on the side.

Add ingredients to a bowl and combine until no lumps.

Pour batter into ramekin.

Microwave for 1 minute on HIGH.

Slice in half and serve.

Enjoy!

Nutrition:

Total

Carbs: 5.4

Fiber: 2g

Protein: 7.3g

Sodium 8%

Hearty Almond Bread

Servings: 8

Preparation Time: 15 minutes

Cooking Time: 60 minutes

Ingredients:

3 cups almond flour

1 teaspoon baking soda

2 teaspoons baking powder

¼ teaspoon sunflower seeds

¼ cup almond milk

½ cup + 2 tablespoons olive oil

3 whole eggs

Directions:

Pre-heat your oven to 300 degrees F.

Take a 9x5 inch loaf pan and grease, keep it on the side.

Add listed ingredients to a bowl and pour the batter into the loaf pan.

Bake for 60 minutes.

Once baked, remove from oven and let it cool.

Slice and serve!

Nutrition:

Calories: 277

Fat: 21g

Carbohydrates: 7g

Protein: 10g ; Sodium 23%

CPSIA information can be obtained
at www.ICGtesting.com
Printed in the USA
BVHW040631260321
603504BV00009B/443

9 781802 086218